Dysautonomia POTS Syndrome

All You Need To Know About Dysautonomia Or POTS Syndrome, All The Symptoms, How To Diagnose POTS Syndrome And The Best Natural And Easy Treatments For Dysautonomia

Mike Mohebbi

If you want to know the latest news and cures about

Dysautonomia POTS Syndrome

Please Visit my Facebook page at:

Http://www.facebook.com/PotsSyndromeDysautonomia

Disclaimer

This book is not intended as a substitute for the medical advice of physicians. The reader should regularly consult a physician in matters relating to his/her health and particularly with respect to any symptoms that may require diagnosis or medical attention.

Table of contents:

Chapter 1: What is POTS Syndrome Dysautonomia: Introduction

Postural Orthostatic Tachycardia Syndrome (POTS) is a rare condition of the heart. This is said to be a condition that occurs in a patient whose heart beat accelerates by more than 30 beats per minute after standing for 10 minutes, without any change in the blood pressure. POTS Syndrome Disease is not very well known even though a lot of people suffer from its symptoms. This disease is also known as POTS Syndrome Dysautonomia or postural tachycardia syndrome.

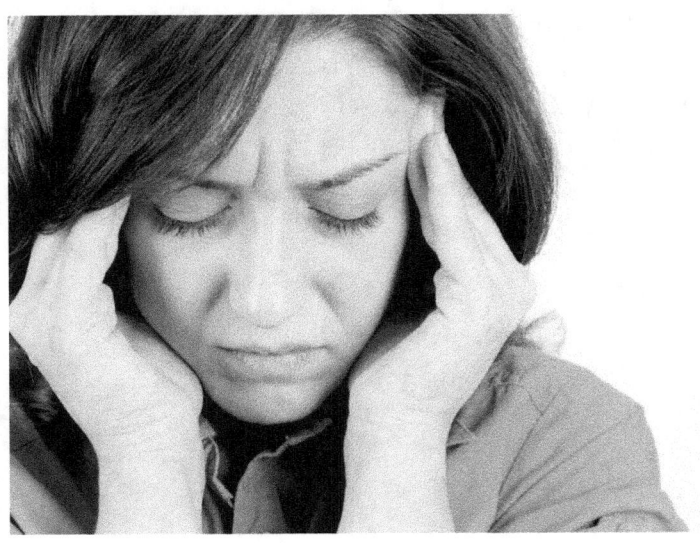

POTS Syndrome Dysautonomia is not life-threatening. The problem with POTS is that its symptoms are almost invisible and also cannot easily be separated from other illnesses having similar symptoms.

Majority of the people with POTS are affected very mildly and only a few develop the severity that can disable them or make them unable to go for work or attend school. What exactly causes POTS is also not known.

How can you distinguish POTS symptoms from normal symptoms?

When you stand up normally, your blood pressure drops slightly as your blood rushes to the belly and tips of our hands and feet due to gravity. Your body responds in the following way: the blood vessels narrow to increase the blood pressure and flow of blood upwards to the heart and brain.

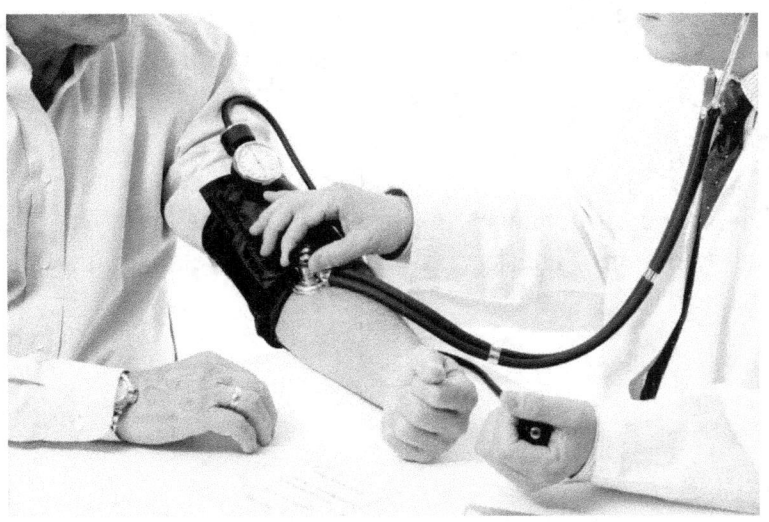

This process of maintaining the blood pressure is automatically done as per the instructions sent by the body's autonomic nervous system.

Most patients who suffer from POTS become easily fatigued, tend to feel dizzy from the lack of sufficient oxygen in the system and can even faint. Associated conditions like sweating and the lack of concentration can make the patient suffer for up to six months.

Is it possible that you may have POTS?

90% people with POTS have mild symptoms that can be managed with changes in lifestyle. A lot of times these

POTS Syndrome Dysautonomia, the pressure does not fall. Anyone feeling these symptoms should see a physician immediately for a checkup and make sure that this is not due to POTS.

There is no specific medication for POTS Syndrome Disease except changes in lifestyle to reduce the effects of the symptoms. The same is discussed in detail in another chapter.

Causes

What causes this problem of the autonomic nervous system remains unexplained. It is seen in young teenagers following a growth spurt, after which the symptoms gradually subside.

It can affect anyone between 15 and 50, with women being most affected.

POTS Syndrome Disease is an illness that can affect one at any time and has been most seen to appear after a:

- Viral attack
- Traumatic event
- Pregnancy
-

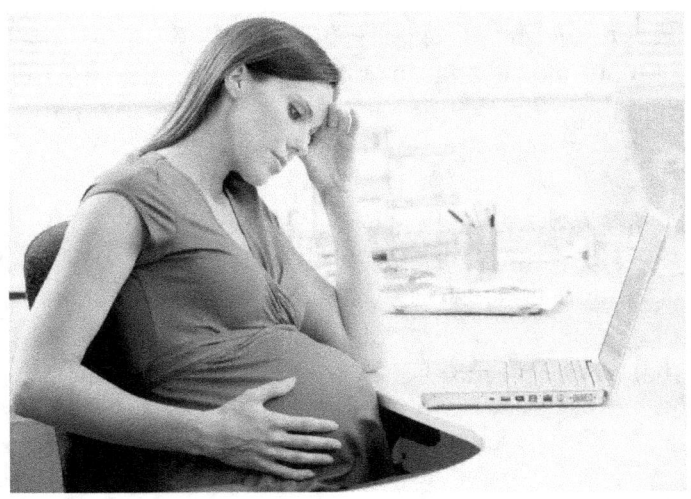

- Joint hyper mobility syndrome –
  - Supple joints
  - Abnormally elastic blood vessels
  - These conditions are often inherited
- Diseases – for example, diabetes and cancer
- Alcohol or metal poisoning
- Inherited condition that produces too much or too little of noradrenalin

As the symptoms can be easily mixed up with other conditions like chronic fatigue syndrome or anxiety attacks, the physician will cross check using appropriate tests to avoid the risk of misdiagnosis.

How is POTS Syndrome Dysautonomia Diagnosed?

When the heart speeds up by 30-40 beats per minute without any change in blood pressure after 10 minutes of standing, it is said to be POTS. The heart rate can be as high as 120 bpm.

When you visit your physician to be treated, many different types of tests will be done to ascertain if the racing heart condition is due to POTS. Please read the chapter for the diagnosis of POTS syndrome to learn more about the tests that can be performed for confirming the diagnosis.

Is it possible to manage the symptoms in the absence of adequate drugs?

The best way to manage POTS symptoms is to closely follow the advice of your physician. In the prescribed list of remedies, you will find a lot of items that are common and well known home remedies. Then, there are those remedies that are a part of a healthy lifestyle.

This is advantageous over taking drugs as the home remedies are natural and you can easily understand what the doctor is asking you to do. Those items on the list that aren't intuitive can easily be incorporated by making small adjustments in your existing life style.

You may also be advised to increase your daily salt intake provided you do not have high blood pressure and a heart condition.

If you have a sudden attack of POTS, lie down and raise your legs and drink at least two glasses of water to lower the heart rate as an emergency measure. Make sure you don't overlook the problem and visit your physician for medical help especially if this is happening for the first time. There are many such small tips that can come in handy while living with POTS. They are discussed in detail in next chapters.

In most cases, patients suffering from POTS Syndrome Dysautonomia will have symptoms that are mild and resolve within a short period of time. Ultimately, for most patients, the symptoms will subside and go away. For those patients having severs symptoms, the time for recovery may be longer with no possibility of recovery.

Hypovolemia and POTS

Hypovolemia is a disorder that reduces the quantity of blood plasma. This unhealthy decrease in the blood sometimes happens in patients having POTS. This is said to occur due to the blood pooling in the abdomen and legs.

The effects of Low Blood Pressure

Having low blood pressure is considered a healthy condition. If standing up causes one's blood pressure to drop suddenly, it leads to a condition known as orthostatic hypotension leading to the symptoms as POTS.

There are a series of clinical conditions that range from fatigue to fainting to over-suppleness of the joints that have symptoms similar to POTS and the doctor will follow similar patterns of treatment as in POTS.

Coping with the symptoms

The treatment for POTS is intimately related to the one's lifestyle and habits. For example; drinking adequately keeps your body hydrated and helps prevent fatigue. The advice is so common place that one may actually overlook it completely. Heat worsens the symptoms and hydration and salt help to maintain body temperature and prevent overheating.

If you have been identified with POTS, then educating yourself about the disease will help you understand that there are many people suffering from it daily and they are able to cope with it successfully. Knowing that you are not alone will lessen your stress.

Understanding the sort of things that can trigger POTS symptoms can also help as a measure of prevention. For example; avoid hot showers and if you must have them, end with a cool one and drink water before and after you shower. Avoid large meals as it makes your digestive system overactive.

Many people worry hearing about POTS. It is an unknown chronic illness which can occur at any time. The symptoms of a pounding heart and chest pains can make you anxious and frightened. If you are over-stressed, you should consider seeing a psychiatrist to talk and seek help on how you can cope with the problem.

If you are unduly frightened, you will only worsen the condition and not be able to use the prescribed advice effectively.

It has been recommended that Cognitive Behavioral Therapy (CBT) can help you cope with your physical limitations given the unpredictability of POTS Syndrome Dysautonomia and its symptoms. CBT will help you adjust to the changes required in your daily routine and keep your attitude positive and confident, which will go a long way in managing this condition effectively.

Chapter 2: What Are the Causes or Risk Factors for POTS Syndrome Dysautonomia?

Postural Orthostatic Tachycardia (POTS Syndrome Disease), also called Postural tachycardia syndrome, is a peculiar disorder, which accelerates the heart beats of the patient during the change in the position of the body. The exact causes of POTS Syndrome Dysautonomia are not known. However, there are some risk factors that can trigger its symptoms or worsen the condition. Patients need to be aware of these symptoms and take proper preventive care with good wellness diet to reduce these symptoms.

Abrupt Increase in Heart Rates

After the meticulous clinical observation and check-ups, doctors confirm the sudden onset of POTS disease to affect the health of the patient. The increment in the diastolic and systolic rates takes a leap from ≥30 to maximum ≥120 bpm without any sign of orthostatic hypotension. When the patient is found lifting his body from supine to the straight/upright position, he actually feels the terrific heart beats. He becomes weak with massive weakness to experience.

More Clinical Tests Needed for Proper Diagnosis

For proper treatment, the patient needs to undergo several clinical trials and blood test to reset the physical functionality. He will have to bring mobility to his body for better movement without hypertension or stress. Within 10 minutes after changing the position to stand firm on the ground, a steady increase in the systolic and diastolic rates by approximately 30 heart beats occurs. Therefore, the patient is seen roaming in frustration with his pale face.

Orthostatic Hypotension Boosts up POTS Syndrome Dysautonomia

Through proper diagnostic procedures and clinical tests, the patients need to be given the medications to tackle the disorder in the heart beats. In this connection, scientists have also done lot of effective researches to detect the causes of POTS disease. In this physical disorder, the tachycardia or fast heart beats are recorded. The orthostatic hypotension takes place because of the abrupt drop in the blood pressure of the affected patient. You will feel a strange lightheadedness, rapid palpitation, discomfort and weakness followed by dyspnea.

Hypovolemia – The Cause of POTS Disease

Researchers have identified certain hidden causes for the recurrent episodes of POTS Syndrome Disease. They reveal some interesting secrets in this regard. They have found that the hypovolemia is the major cause that boosts up the possibilities of the onset of this type of tachycardia.

Decrease in the Blood Flow Speeds up POTS Disease

Experienced medical scientists have stated that the palpable decrease in the channelization of the blood to the heart causes the blood pulling, which results in sudden hypotension. The heart is forced to expand for blood pumping due to such poor blood supply. Hypovolemia is therefore one of the visible causes for the occurrence of the POTS Syndrome Disease.

Abnormality in Cardiac Functionality

Owing to the abnormality in the output of cardiac functionality, it snowballs into pre-syncope with reflex tachycardia. You will have to struggle for the restoration of energy to feel normal with good efficiency to breathe fresh air. You must be dynamic with proper healthcare.

Norepinephrine Level Increases

To be frank, the level of norepinephrine starts bobbing up on account of the hypovolemia. When the heart compensates by beating faster, the patient feels an awkward vision blurring, weakness and breathing disorder. It is due to the faster heart beat with mild automatic neuropathic disorder. On the other hand, during the vast research, scientists have also discovered a prominent acceleration of heart beats even in the absence of low blood flow to the heart. This condition is identified as central hyperadrenergic syndrome. You will have to consult a specialist to change or tailor the regular dietary plan for speedy recuperation from such a pre-existing health problem.

POTS Associated with Fatigue

In spite of an inability to track the exact causes of POTS Syndrome Dysautonomia, experienced researchers have put focus on the involvement of orthostatic intolerance to influence the onset of this severe syndrome. POTS Disease is also associated with some chronic physical disorders like fatigue. The patient loses his strength to have an upright position under the compulsion of this orthostatic intolerance.

Health Condition Deteriorates

When a patient suffers from painful viral infection or prolonged illness, his health condition starts going down. For this reason, slowly, the patient is wondering in the state of hallucination with the least ability to stand boldly. So this physical condition is closely connected with the impact of the POTS disease.

Secondary Syndrome Connected with POTS

Scientists launched more result-oriented surveys probing to unearth the invisible factors that may influence the POTS disease, as they suspected the existence of a secondary syndrome. The presence of diabetes mellitus is an important factor to enhance the rapid deterioration in the health condition of the patient. Gradually, the patient has to undergo severe fatigue and gastrointestinal disorder.

More Prominent Risks

According to leading physicians and researchers in the European POTS research centers, the intake of fluid is affected due to the occurrence of nausea. Additionally, the loss of fluid takes place faster during the diarrhea. Eventually, the patient has to face the hypovolemic disorder. So indirectly, patient experiences the POTS Syndrome Dysautonomia with rapid breakdown in the nervous system. He never gets energy to move freely. His body becomes sturdy with long lasting lightheadedness, nausea and discomfort.

Preventive Care

Patients with POTS Syndrome Dysautonomia must be more cautious. They should have good home-based preventive care and medical assistance to ensure better improvement. That's why; experts have designed cost-effective dietary programs to prevent the risks of being severely bruised by this chronic syndrome. For instance, the regular water intake frequency must gear up for well compensation. The blood flow needs to be increased to check the severity of hypovolemia.

Important Facts

The loss of energy should be stopped. Doctors recommend some home based treatments for the prevention of POTS. Before taking nutrients and any healthcare supplement, you must finish an effective discussion with your home physician for better solution. POTS Syndrome Dysautonomia should be boldly taken care of without negligence. In this regard, online free training and consultation help novice people to know about the side effect, causes and remedies to shrug off the POTS disease.

The online education and healthcare campaigns play a role in training adult people to handle this disease. Doctors have not found any performance specific treatment to wipe out the symptoms of POTS. However, they may prescribe some easy-to-maintain health management and POTS preventive plans to enable patients to recuperate faster. They must take nutritious foods, drink lot of fresh water and do proper wellness exercises to rebuild the body. They have to reinforce their immune system to resist the negative effect of POTS.

Chapter 3: The common signs and symptoms of POTS Syndrome Dysautonomia

People sometimes ask whether the symptoms of Postural Orthostatic Tachycardia Syndrome can be clearly laid down. Well, the answer is no, because **POTS Syndrome Dysautonomia** has symptoms consistent with some other medical conditions. For example, when asked whether having palpitations or a severe headache is a symptom of POTS, doctors, in a majority of cases, are at a loss of words and are not able to give an immediate answer. This is because many of the symptoms of **POTS Syndrome Dysautonomia** are similar to the symptoms of conditions like anxiety and migraine.

POTS disease is often called the invisible disease because it does not present itself openly and is, many times, mistaken to be something else. It takes usually at least two years to reach a conclusive diagnosis of the syndrome.

The main symptoms are very much evident from the name of the disease itself and an attempt has been made here to enumerate them in layman's terms. They are as follows:

- Dizziness on changing posture: This comes from the word Postural Orthostatic. When the patient changes from a sitting position to a standing position, he feels dizzy. He might sometimes even pass out. This is because the blood is not able to reach the brain immediately on standing up, as it usually does for normal people. The affected person feels as if they are going to pass out and so, want to hold on to some kind of support; but in many cases, they do not actually fall down.

- Fatigue: The patient suddenly feels extremely fatigued and is not even able to sit up. He or she just wants to lie down. They might also have weakness, shaking or tremors and bladder dysfunction. They might find it a herculean task even to move from one room to another.

- Racing heart beat: Fast heart beat or Tachycardia is an important symptom of POTS. That is what T stands for in the abbreviation. There is an increase in the heartbeat by up to 30 beats per minute, on change of posture, from sitting to standing or walking.

- Severe headaches: POTS Syndrome Dysautonomia is often characterized by severe headaches which resemble migraines. The patient is affected by bright light and loud noise, which is very similar to migraine. This often leads the physician to make a wrong diagnosis, in the early stages.

  The patient may be affected by the normal sound level of a video game, for example. Hence, they are not able to enjoy the life in the normal way.

- Nausea and abdominal pain: The patient experiences chronic abdominal pain and stomach cramps in many cases. The stomach feels tight and pulled up. This is because the nervous supply to the stomach does not function properly and can result in bloating, diarrhea and constipation. They can also experience chest pains in some cases. The patient also feels a vomiting sensation and does not like to eat anything for the fear of throwing up. Immediately after eating, they might want to use the restroom a number of times because of the abdominal discomfort.

- Palpitations and chest pains: palpitations are a result of the racing heart and the patient feels short of breath. They feel as if the lung is constricted and have difficulty in breathing. They may also feel severe lower back pain and it sometimes seems to be shifting from one place to another.

- Sleep Apnea: the patient may experience lack of sleep or insomnia. Another symptom of POTS Syndrome Dysautonomia is sleep apnea, where they feel breathlessness in mid sleep.

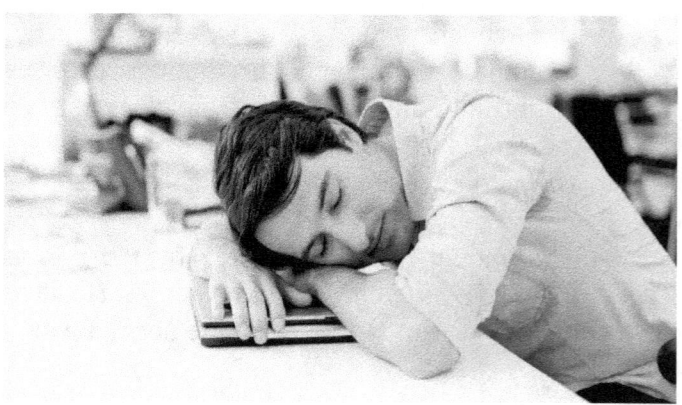

- Sweating abnormally: there are reports of extreme sweating in some cases. The patient sweats profusely as a result of the fast heartbeat.

- Brain Fog: many patients find it difficult to focus and concentrate. Their communication ability is also impaired. Therefore, sometimes they are not able to continue their studies or attend work. They may experience a little memory loss too, like suddenly forgetting the notes of a song midway.

- Bluish or reddish legs: this happens because of the blood pooling in the lower parts of the body, particularly the legs. The blood vessels do not constrict and help the blood to flow to the upper parts of the body. There is, however, no problem with the normal functioning of the legs. Only the appearance of the leg is different, usually on standing up.

The above mentioned symptoms are the physical indicators of POTS Syndrome Disease. In addition, there are some psychological symptoms too, which have to be taken into account.

The person feels overly stressed and therefore gets angry and depressed. They may also be anxious about their next fainting episode. This makes them nervous and disturbed. They need to sleep and rest a lot and this interferes with their daily life. They feel tired and drained out for almost the entire day. However, suddenly there might be some good days when they feel like they can take up some simple activities. These symptoms look very similar to the signs of anxiety or depression; but they are the indications of POTS.

People afflicted by Dysautonomia, are affected by change in temperature. So, an increase in heat brings in more weariness and worsens the tachycardia.

If patients experience any of these symptoms, they should consult a doctor to confirm or rule out the diagnosis of the

POTS Syndrome Dysautonomia rather than trying any self-medication.

Chapter 4: Different diagnostic methods used for detecting a POTS Syndrome Dysautonomia

In this chapter, you will find methods and techniques used for POTS Syndrome Dysautonomia detection. These diagnostic methods are broadly classified as preliminary tests or symptoms, initial investigations and finally disease specific investigations. Usually, the preliminary tests indicate whether further investigations are necessary or not. Many of these preliminary tests can also be done at home because there are diagnostic instruments that are now available that you can use yourself at homes.

Symptoms or Preliminary Tests for Diagnosing POTS Syndrome Dysautonomia that a doctor may ask you before confirming the diagnosis:

1. Do you feel lightheaded?
2. Do you feel your heart is beating rapidly or do you feel any chest pain?
3. Active Stand Test-
   Does your heart start beating at a very high rate when you are standing for long, i.e., 5 to 30 minutes? This test is called the Active Stand Test. You can check your heart rate in the resting position

and then as you stand up. After waiting for 2 minutes and then 5 minutes, you can check your heartbeat.

4. Do you have an intolerance to exercise?
5. Do you suffer from a headache at such times?
6. Do you feel extremely tired at such times?
7. Do you feel as if you may faint or feel like vomiting? Alternatively, are you suffering from diarrhea?
8. Do you feel shaky when you stand?
9. Do you experience excess sweating or bladder problems?
10. Do you have a problem in concentrating?
11. Has your sleep pattern undergone change or are you sleeping less?
12. Do you have a problem with your vision?
13. Do you feel very thirsty and in general, frequently dehydrated?
14. Do you notice these symptoms when you are getting up, standing up suddenly, have finished eating or are living in hot conditions?
15. Is your heart rate normal when you lie down?

Initial Investigations

If you have the symptoms mentioned above, you can undergo for further investigations for the diagnosis of POTS Syndrome Disease.

1. Tilting the Head Up

This test is usually performed by the doctor. The doctor uses a table to lift your head up to about 60 degrees or slightly more. The doctor may also dim the light in the room. The temperature of the room will be maintained steadily and your blood pressure, as well as heart beats, will be noted from the position when you were resting on the flat table to the tilted position. If you do have POTS Syndrome Dysautonomia, your heart rate will exceed by 30 beats per minute within 10 minutes or so. Some POTS patients, however, may reveal such heart beat variation much later, i.e., when such tilted position is maintained for 45 minutes.

2. Monitoring heart rate and blood pressure

using ambulatory monitoring devices. Sticky patches can be attached to different parts of your chest and recordings for an entire day will be taken in a small box which can be carried around.

3. ECG

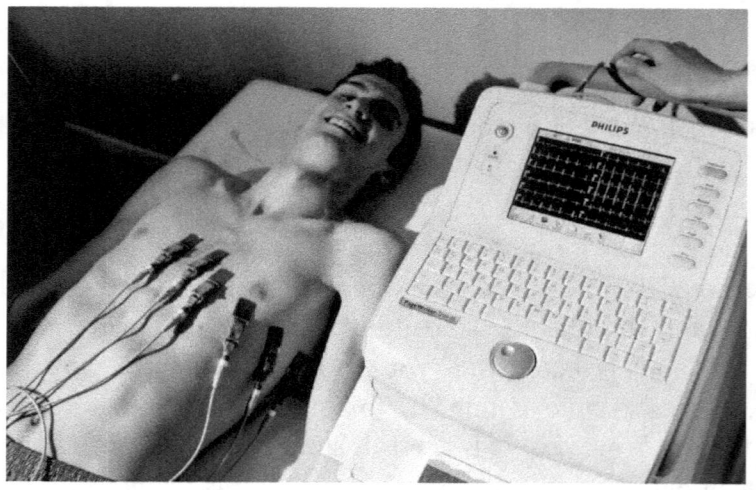

This is a test with which almost everybody who knows something about the heart is familiar with. This test will reveal if your heart is behaving abnormally or has behaved abnormally in recent past.

4. Echocardiogram (Heart Ultrasound)

Like ECG, this test is for getting some information about your heart; but as a three-dimensional picture.

5. Cold Presser

This test is used to find out changes in the blood pressure due to the changes in conditions. You will be asked to place your hands in cold water and your physician will measure the changes in your blood pressure.

6. Paced Respiration and Deep Breathing

Your physician will ask you to breathe at a specific pace and measure your heartbeat and blood pressure. Similarly, your physician may ask you to take a deep breath and then measure your heart beat as well as blood pressure.

7. Hand Grip Test

For this test, your physician will ask you to press something with your hand, more specifically within your grip, until you are tired.

8. Baroreflex

This is a blowing machine in which you will have to blow the balloons. It will indicate when you are feeling weak. You may get a headache and your blood pressure may increase with such a tool.

9. Stress Test

This will indicate how your heart is functioning under the stress conditions.

Disease-Specific Investigations

These detailed investigations are performed for the final diagnosis of **POTS Syndrome Disease.**

1. **Transcranial Doppler Ultrasonography** – This test will indicate the amount of blood supply that is reaching your brain. The blood flow will be less than 2000 in the case of POTS patients.

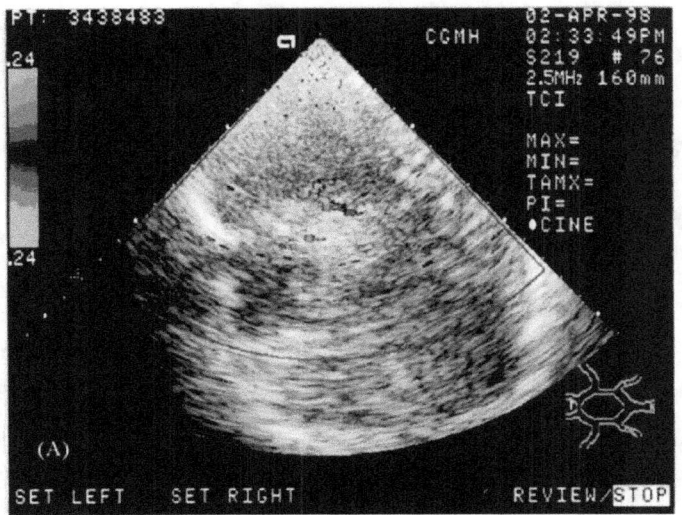

2. **Bowel Motility Studies** – The studies help in finding out to what extent your gastrointestinal system is contributing to such increase in the heart rate.

3. **Urine Tests for Sodium** – These tests are done on urine for two consecutive days with a gap not exceeding 24 hours. If you have POTS, your urine will have rather a low amount of sodium in it, i.e., less than 150 mill moles. However, similar symptoms are also possible if your urine has high levels of epinephrine or noradrenaline. Any growth on your adrenaline gland can also result in an increase in these two hormones or neurotransmitters. Therefore, you physician will test your urine after another 24 hours as well for determining the most specific cause.

4. **Catecholamine Test-** This test is usually done for detecting tumors, but some patients with POTS Syndrome Dysautonomia also show the unusually high level of this plasma protein and other plasma proteins such as norepinephrine. These proteins increase because of fear, which is normally associated with tachycardia, i.e., rapid beating of your heart.

5. **MRI** – You may be asked to undergo this test because this test is used to indicate tumors, cervical stenosis, Chiari or other diseases.

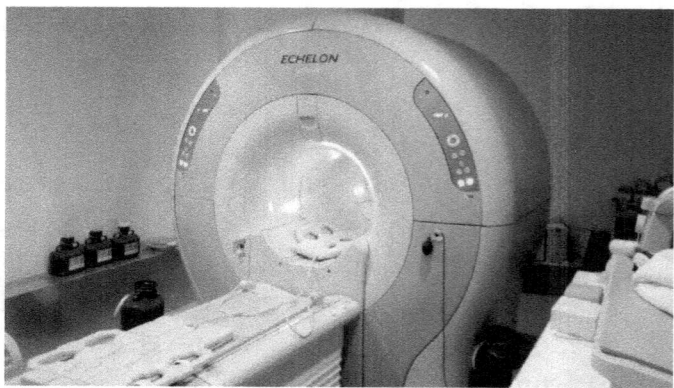

Symptoms of such ailments resemble those of POTS disease. If these tests prove negative, then possibility of you having POTS Syndrome Dysautonomia increases.

6. **Blood Tests** – These are necessary to rule out problems with your liver, kidney, thyroid, glucose levels, calcium levels and in general, the blood count. Hypovolemia may at times be found along with POTS. Therefore, plasma volume, as well as the mass of red cells, becomes important.

7. **Electromyography and Microneurography-** In these tests, your nervous system is checked to rule out that problem. In microneurography, a needle placed inside the leg indicates how the signals from the nervous system are traveling.

8. **Autonomic Function Testing** – These tests check how your peripheral and central nervous system are functioning. The tests include Sweat testing or QSART, which is a test for nerves that control your sweating function, apart from TST or Thermoregulatory Sweat Test and QST or Quantitative Sensory Test. The thermoregulatory sweat test indicates the ability of the body to produce sweat for regulating the body temperature and the QST is for sensing temperature or vibrations.

As can be seen from above, that positive results for POTS Syndrome Dysautonomia from most of the diagnostic tests under first two categories would make necessary that the last category tests should be performed. Some of these tests such as MRI are essentially for ruling out some possibilities. Therefore, you should not panic as it can increase your catecholamine and lead to a wrong diagnosis.

Chapter 5: What can be the complications of POTS Syndrome Dysautonomia?

POTS Syndrome Dysautonomia is being looked upon as a debilitating and altering health condition. Those suffering from this disease find it challenging even to stand straight. This is because of the body's inability to adjust with the gravitational force.

As discussed earlier, the main characteristic that highlights POTS disease is orthostatic intolerance along with the symptoms like fatigue, headaches, palpitations, nausea, sweating, dizziness and fainting. Adding further, the rate of heart beat also increases while in upright position.

Complications Associated with POTS Dysautonomia

Patients and strangely, even the medical professionals have misconceptions about POTS. Although less popular, it is not a rare disease. The patients suffering from POTS Syndrome Disease have to struggle a lot because of the disabling and unpredictable traits associated.

POTS disease is considered as a spectrum. Many people find it hard to believe that one can live actively with the disease. However, it is a misconception. Although there are waxing and waning symptoms that come and go, patients lead fairly normal lives. But, this doesn't imply that POTS disease is easy to live or deal with.

POTS disease is not deadly by itself; but the associated complications can be risky. As the name implies, POTS Syndrome Dysautonomia, is a collection of symptoms and not a disease by itself. Have a look at the following complications associated with the POTS disease and the ways to deal with them.

- **Orthostatic Intolerance**

Orthostatic Intolerance is a health condition wherein the patient experiences remarkably reduced volume of blood returning to the heart on getting back to an upright position from the lying down position. These complications are further accompanied by a rapid increase in the heart rate, by about 30 or more beats per minute.

Putting it other way, the person experiences a heart rate in excess of 120 beats a minute within a span of about 10 minutes from standing up. This condition can be relieved by returning to the lying down position. Due to this, the patient may feel overtly anxious and faces a danger of doing activities that can cause harm.

- **Lightheadedness or fainting**

POTS can attack any age group, specifically women between age of 15 and 50 years. This condition is characterized by feelings like fainting or lightheadedness. The syndrome has also shown people's inability to exercise because of prompt fainting and dizziness. There is always a danger of falling or tripping while working on a treadmill, jogging and cycling resulting in accidents.

Some other complications associated with POTS Syndrome Dysautonomia include:

- **Irritable Bowel Syndrome**

Irritable Bowel Syndrome, or IBS, refers to a functional disorder associated with large intestine. The effects of IBS usually vary from constipation to diarrhea.

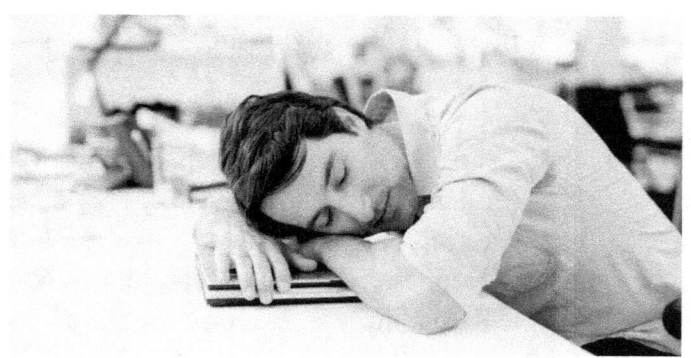

Many of you might experience mucus in the stool, while others might feel like having another bowel movement just after you have had one. You might also experience bloating, gas and cramping, all of these being painful symptoms that cause inconvenience and discomfort. Although chronic, the symptoms of IBS can vary over time.

These IBS symptoms can be reduced through general precautions. Usually, foods like carbonated beverages, alcohol, caffeine, chocolates, milk products and fatty foods trigger the symptoms of IBS. Try to find the culprit and eliminate it from your diet to ease the condition.

Another way to reduce the symptoms of IBS is to include natural fiber in your diet by consuming more fruits and vegetables. However, over consumption of fiber might end up in creating more gas in the stomach thereby further irritating the stomach even more.

Some other intestinal disorders may also occur with similar symptoms. It is; therefore, wise to consult a doctor in time rather than relying solely on all sorts of information floating through the internet.

- **Restless Leg Syndrome**

Another complication associated with the POTS Syndrome Dysautonomia is Restless Leg Syndrome (RLS). It refers to a disorder associated with the nervous system. It generally affects the leg movement. This condition is also considered a neurological sleep disorder that interferes with the normal sleep.

This condition is characterized by extreme discomfort in legs while sitting and lying. You might feel like getting up and move around. Doing so would relieve you from the discomfort and the unpleasant feeling of restlessness.

Although movement of legs can provide temporary relief from the condition, doctors recommend certain lifestyle changes along with certain activities to relieve the symptoms like itching, creeping, creepy crawly, pulling, gnawing or tugging.

Lowering the intake of alcohol, caffeine, and tobacco can also be helpful.

- **Dysautonomia**

"Dysautonomia" is a term used to refer to numerous medical conditions   that lead to the malfunctioning of your autonomic nervous system. The autonomic nervous system is responsible for controlling the sub-conscious nervous activities like blood pressure, digestion, heart rate, dilation and constriction of the pupils, kidney function and temperature control.

- **Chronic Fatigue Syndrome**

The Chronic Fatigue Syndrome is a condition that refers to a complicated disorder with symptoms like extreme fatigue.   The condition doesn't improve even with extreme bed rest. Instead, it worsens with mental or physical activity.

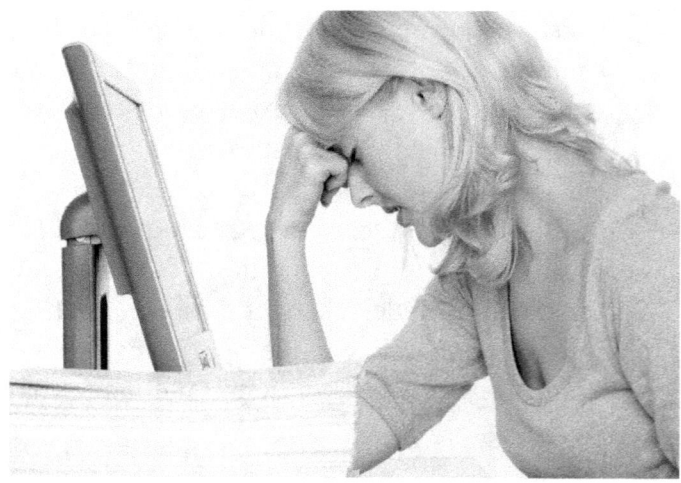

The key symptoms of Chronic Fatigue Syndrome include cognitive difficulties, muscle and joint pain and severe physical and mental exhaustion.

Chronic or severe fatigue that has lasted for over 6 months cannot be reduced by rest. Generally, treatments recommended by doctors include diets, supplements, physiotherapy, anti-depressants, pacing, energy management, pain killers, graded activity/exercise and alternative or complementary medication.

The therapies recommended by doctors for POTS Syndrome Dysautonomia aim at relieving the low volume of blood or regulating the circulatory issues resulting from the disease. The treatment options vary for different individuals, depending upon the physical conditions and the intensity of complications.

The POTS Syndrome Dysautonomia can lead to a relapsing-remitting condition wherein the symptoms might come and go over span of time. In majority of cases, the patients improve even after associated complications. However, in case of more intense complications, the patients might get bed ridden for life or not improve or recover at a desirable pace. The recovery depends upon the severity of the complications and treatment provided. A regular treatment and some simple precautions can help in preventing most of these complications. Hence, it is very important that you consult your doctor and take timely treatment for this condition.

Chapter 6: The foods to be eaten and avoided by patients with POTS Syndrome Dysautonomia

'POTS' is not actually a disease, which is why it is known as a Syndrome. There are certain reasons for the occurrence of this condition. However, the symptoms of POTS Syndrome Dysautonomia and the complications that may arise due to it can be prevented through consuming and avoiding certain food. However, no matter whether you have POTS or not, you must take care of your health, by consuming healthy food, and avoiding unhealthy Foods.

Some of the food that can be consumed is the fluids such as water, green juice, soups, lemon juice, cucumber and tomato salads and cereals with salt sprinkled on it. Whole grain and fruit should also be eaten in plenty. Avoid food items which have gluten, as it results in neurological disorders. Sugar-rich food and white flour must be avoided, even dairy and junk foods must be prohibited and besides these, you should also stop consuming energy drinks to maintain good health.

Intake of Salt is Important

Salt is found to be more effective in the treatment of POTS Syndrome Dysautonomia, and is highly recommended by the physicians. If you cannot consume salt directly, you can use it in various ways. You can sprinkle salt and lemon on all the foods that you eat. This not only increases the taste of the food, but also improves your health protecting you from POTS. But, avoid salt usage if you have any heart or kidney problems. You can also choose to drink half a cup of salt water for at least twice a week.

Intake of Water and Soup

Intake of water is also utmost important, similar to salt consumption. You have to consume plenty of water (for about a glass per 15 minutes). This will keep your body cool and thereby relax your mind. Higher amount of water consumption is found to be beneficial for the POTS patients. It leads to the improvements in standing blood pressure and heart rate. Even, soup can be consumed, which offers same benefit as that of the water. Drink healthy soups with plenty of vegetables to maintain good health.

Green Juice for Better Health

Green Juice can be prepared in various ways using different vegetables and fruits. You can prepare green juice by using spinach, vegetables, cereals and dry fruits. Either you can make this juice sweet or salty and spicy. However, it's better to consume green juice by adding little bit of salt. But do make it spicy by adding all spicy items. To sweeten don't use sugar, instead use honey which is good for your health. Drink it during your breakfast time to strengthen and energize your body as well as to keep yourself active all the day.

Eat Fresh fruits and Vegetables

You can consume fresh fruits and vegetables like cucumber, tomatoes, bitter gourd and others. Best method is to have cucumbers and tomatoes in the form of Salads. You need to cut tomatoes and cucumbers in a circular way or into small pieces, then sprinkle some salt over it and consume. As simple as that! Ensure that, the tomatoes and cucumbers are fresh. Besides these, you can have bitter gourd, which is extremely good for your health, though it tastes bitter. You can cut bitter gourd, put the pieces in a pan, pour few spoons of oil and heat in a low frame. Later, you can sprinkle salt over these and consume it with brown bread. Also, you can have raw Spinach in your lunch and dinner, along with other cooked food.

Avoid Energy Drinks

Because of weakness, many people drink milk, while some use Energy drinks to become much strong. This is a wrong idea if you want to become strong.

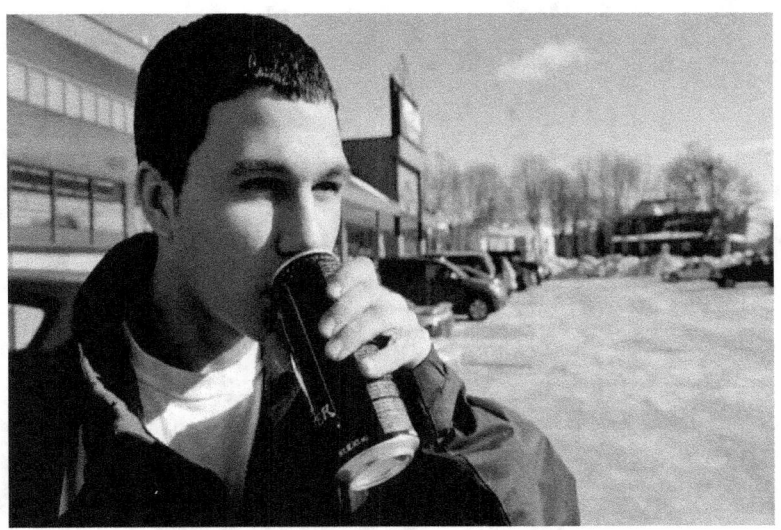

Drinking Milk is okay to some extent, but not the Energy Drinks. These Energy drinks typically include Caffeine as well as Guarana. In fact, Caffeine may worsen the symptoms of POTS in few patients.

Avoid Gluten and Dairy

As per the symptoms found, people can try some food combination as well as avoid certain foods to check how they can reduce POTS Syndrome Dysautonomia. One of such experiment includes avoiding Gluten and Dairy products. Consuming more amounts of Gluten and dairy products can often worsen the situation. Therefore, if you are suffering from POTS, avoid the intake of these Gluten and Dairy products to see the positive results.

Avoid Large Meals

Some people make it a habit to eat large meals in a single time, which really worsens the symptoms of POTS. Researchers have also found that, patients with this problem usually have post-prandial hypotension. This is a low blood pressure, which makes one feel dizzy or faint. This critical condition is caused due to the blood pooling in the abdominal area. And it usually happens when food is digested.

That means, if more food is consumed at a time, you will be in need of more blood to digest the food properly. But, when more blood is used to digest the food, you feel dizzy. Hence, doctors advise the patients to eat less or minimal amounts of food, but increase the number of times you eat the food throughout the day.

Therefore, consume less food and avoid the consumption of large meals. This, in turn, will help you to avoid the disturbing symptoms of POTS.

Avoid Junk Food

Junk food must be prohibited. It will only spoil your health further! Consumption of junk foods like cakes, pizzas, burgers, pasta, noodles, etc., may increase the symptoms of POTS and make you suffer more.

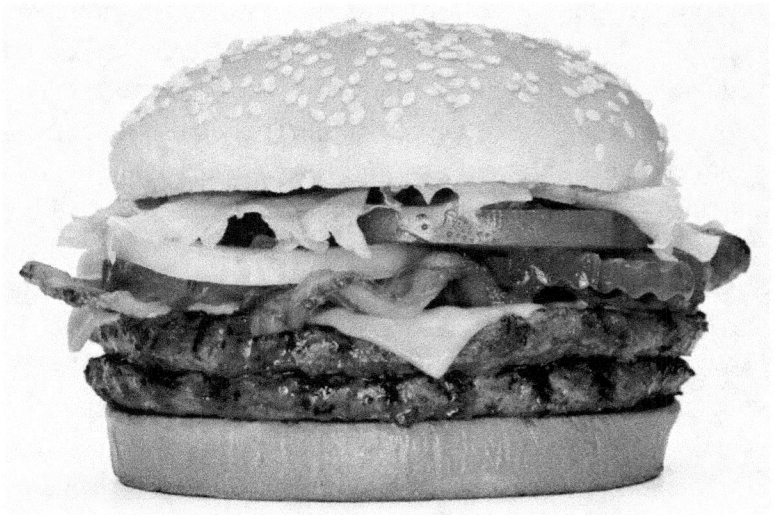

These junk foods contain worst chemicals such as the artificial food colors and flavors, which affect your health adversely. Hence, avoid these junk food and practice eating nutritious food. Some people may go for vitamin and nutrition supplements that arrive in the form of pills, tablets, powder or syrup. But, when you have to make a choice between natural nutritious foods and artificial supplementary tablets, it's the natural food that wins the race to a healthy life. So go with natural foods. Eat more amounts of green veggies, various types of fruits and so on. By consuming these, your body will get enough amounts of potassium, magnesium and calcium that keep you healthy all the times.

Avoid Non-Vegetarian Food and Alcohol

If you are getting lots of vitamins, minerals, nutrition, Omega-3 fatty acids and so on in different types of vegetables, why do you prefer non-vegetarian food? You know something? People consuming vegetables are much stronger than the people eating non-vegetarian food. You can just think of elephant. Elephant eats grass and other green leafy vegetables, fruits, etc. Is elephant weaker than any other wild animal? It is quite larger than other animals and also stronger. Therefore, to remain healthy like an elephant, always consume vegetarian food and avoid non-vegetarian food. Eating fresh vegetables and fruits can actually keep you calm and make you more active. But, non-vegetarian food can create more disturbing symptoms including indigestion and anxiety inside you. You may eat non-vegetarian food once or twice in a month, but not on a regular basis.

Another thing that has to be avoided is the drugs. Throw away all your bad habits like drinking alcohol, smoking and any other you may have. This will definitely help you to stay away from POTS.

Chapter 7: Alternative modes of treatment for POTS Syndrome Dysautonomia

Seeing the widespread effects of POTS Syndrome Dysautonomia, the need of the hour is to look for the alternative treatment modes for the same. In this chapter, you will get to know the various therapies, which will help cure this disease of yours! Well, don't be afraid of **the POTS Syndrome Disease**, for now the science is much advanced and developed. Just have a look on the below mentioned therapies.

Well, exercise is the first medicine to very disease. According to a recent survey, The POTS disease can be healed without any drugs or surgery, if the patient wishes to and shows full dedication towards the same. You can take the guidance of a health expert and he can guide you with what type of exercises to carry on and what not. Mostly the sitting exercises are preferred to get over this disease. Just go for a regular exercise schedule and see the drastic changes yourself and be amazed!

To go for a more scientific approach, there are a number of therapies to cure the POTS Syndrome Disease.

Acupressure:

Very simple to carry out! Just use your finger tips on some of the body parts and press a bit harder. It helps you to get rid of all the pains and aches and help you feel much relaxed and happy. Thus, it also reduces the chances of any heart disease. Acupressure has proved to be of really great help to the POTS Syndrome Dysautonomia patients.

Acupuncture

Acupuncture is done with the use of fine needles. They are inserted at some specific points along the body to regulate the proper flow of energy and blood, so that no clotting or any such problem arises. Along with the balanced energy level, acupuncture also helps to cure the degenerative problems among the children as well as the old aged ones.

Ayurvedic Medicine

As goes the saying' 'Old is Gold"! The Ayurvedic treatment exists in India from around 5000 hundred years ago and has shown its effect in almost every field of healthcare. It focuses on the natural treatment and helps you avoid the intake of the allopathic medicines that are known to cause too many side effects. Just simple tongue testing and checking the pulse can let an Ayurvedic physician know a lot about the physical illness of the patient, if done at an initial stage. The POTS Syndrome

Dysautonomia can also be cured with the use of the Ayurvedic medicines.

Auricular Therapy

Well, according to the old Egyptian beliefs, a person can be relieved from pain up to a great extent by the Auricular Therapy. As per this, specific parts of the ear need to be massaged and it really works for the POTS Syndrome Dysautonomia as well.

Chiropractic

Doctors' worldwide suggest the Chiropractic therapy to be one of the best cures for the POTS Syndrome Disease. Try this out and see the results yourself.

The above-mentioned therapies are of great help to the people, if they take it seriously. Mostly it is seen that patients have a set thinking that this disease cannot be cured at any cost, which is wrong.

Always remember that the POTS Syndrome Dysautonomia can only be cured if you think it can be cured! Apart from all these therapies, as said earlier, exercise should be the foremost priority. It provides you an alert lifestyle and fills you with energy and vitality. All your body parts come into action and you start feeling fresher day by day. The blood flow is regulated in a correct manner and the nervous system also works just perfectly. Engage yourself in moderate and upright position exercises such as cycling, biking, riding and so on, whichever gives you the best comfort level.

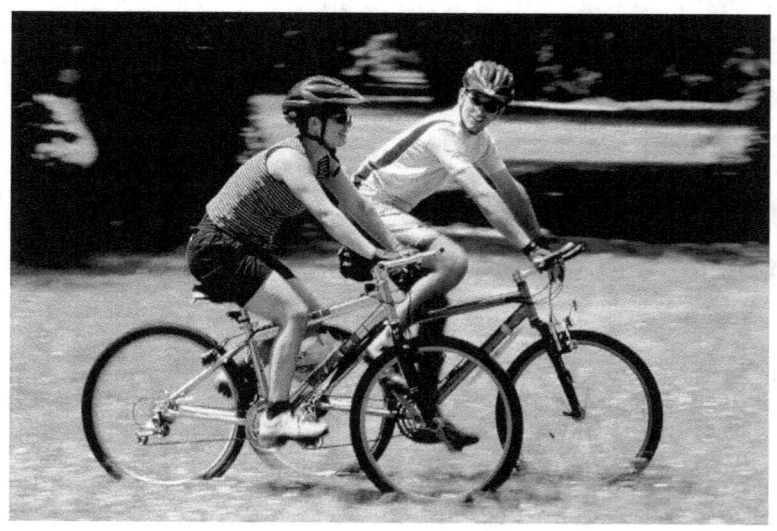

Do take the advice of a health expert before starting anything and I am sure that your POTS Syndrome Disease will be cured easily, without taking any expensive treatment. According to a recent survey, the percentage of people who were cured of the POTS Syndrome Dysautonomia by just regularly exercising was 25% more than the ones who went for surgeries or any other treatment.

The statistical figures are in itself a proof of what should be done and what not. The decision lies in your hands, for you are the master of your own health!

Also, the patients of POTS Syndrome Disease should keep a check on their diet as well. They should avoid the oily food as much as possible and prefer green vegetables. Besides this, a lot of water should be added in your daily diet.

Water is very essential as it helps clear your immune system up to a great extent, which is very important.

You may also go for physiological counseling to get rid of the side effects of the POTS Syndrome Disease like anxiety, depression and many other complicating factors.

In this chapter, we studied how the POTS Syndrome Dysautonomia can be cured using the alternative modes of therapies. Also, we came across the role of exercise and diet in the healing of this disease.

If you have a strong determination and will-power, you can easily overcome this disease, no matter what. It will take time and a lot of effort at least initially; but then the results will be worth it. Though the process may be very time consuming, do not lose your calm, for it is you who has to get over this disease.

Chapter 8: Simple Tips And Strategies To Obtain Relief From POTS Syndrome Dysautonomia

Living with POTS disease syndrome can be difficult. However, following some simple tips and the use of some herbs can make it easier for you to gain control over the disease. Here are some time-tested strategies that will help you obtain relief from the disturbing symptoms of POTS disease.

Ginger

Nausea is one of the most troublesome symptoms of POTS disease. Ginger can be used in several different ways to control this symptom. You can say it is a lifesaver! You can add grated ginger to your lemon tea and brew it for about 5 minutes. Drink it to obtain instant relief from nausea and to feel refreshed. You can also add ginger to the dishes you prepare to keep the symptom at bay.

Vitamin D

It has been found that vitamin D helps to ease the symptoms of POTS disease. Sunlight is the best natural source for vitamin D. Patients are advised to spend at least

30 minutes outdoors every day so that they get sufficient amount of sunlight, which enables the body to produce vitamin D. The best way to do this is to park your car 4 blocks away from your office and then take a walk to and from your workplace.

Wear Good Sunglasses

Though sunrays can be good for you in your fight against POTS disease, it may cause harm to your eyes and also increase your sensitivity to light. Hence, it is as important to wear good sunglasses to block the harmful UV rays as it is to go out in the sun to get your dose of vitamin D. This is especially true for those having sensitivity to bright light.

Pistachio And Pomegranate

Pistachio and pomegranate are not just palatable for your taste buds, but also the best natural fighters against POTS disease. They can help by boosting your blood-making process and also improve your immunity. These fruits also provide a very good source of vitamins for the body.

Meditation And Positive Thinking

Meditation can pave the way for a healthier and happier life and help you gain control over the symptoms of POTS disease. Meditation boosts positive thinking and allows you to be optimistic about the outcome of the treatment. This may seem too theoretic; however, most patients gain miraculous results with meditation and positive thinking.

It also allows you to concentrate on the things you can do and accept the things that you can't. This makes you happier and satisfied with what you have.

These tips seem very simple; however, they can make a lot of difference to your life by easing your symptoms. Follow these tips and make them a part of your routine to get rid of the annoying symptoms of POTS disease and to improve the quality of your life.

Chapter 8: Conclusion

Living with POTS: What types of adjustments are required to make every day easier!

People with POTS Syndrome Dysautonomia might appear to be just fine, while they actually feel very sick inside. It is a very debilitating condition, which can possibly put patients in a wheel chair permanently, simply because they do not have the strength to stand up on their legs. Sometimes, people diagnosed with POTS might need frequent hospital visits to keep the condition under control. Most people are also worried that they are suffering from some deadly disease. However, this is not true. It is very easy to live a comfortable and long life even when you are suffering from POTS disease. All you need to do is follow some simple precautions and make few changes to your lifestyle!

Even today, nearly 20 years after the condition was first identified and categorized, it takes long time to diagnose this autoimmune disorder. The symptoms are similar to a lot of other medical conditions like anxiety and vertigo. Furthermore, they are extremely varied and change on a day to day basis. Therefore, while it is not easy to live with POTS Syndrome Dysautonomia, there are some tips, which can make life with the condition easier. Here is a brief summary of some of the most important points that will help you live a comfortable and independent life.

As discussed earlier, drinking a lot of water can be good for the person affected by the syndrome, to drink lots of water and keep hydrated. However, consuming sugary drinks is not good. It is good to have smart water and seltzer water. You can drink tomato juice adding salt to it or a mixed veggie juice with salt.

Intake of salt is also a very important factor for people with POTS. It gives you a lot of energy. You can sprinkle salt on watermelon or apple pieces and have them. Strawberries and cantaloupes also taste good, along with a pinch of salt. If you have high blood pressure, then please monitor your blood pressure levels while increasing your salt intake. But generally people with POTS have low B.P. It is good to take a lot of soup.

Also, make sure you avoid drinking sugary caffeinated drinks like Coco-Cola. Soda and sugar will surely increase the tachycardia and that is bad.

It is good for you to do moderate exercise while using a heart rate monitor. Exercises in sitting position, where the head is as close to the leg as possible are good. It is very beneficial to do swimming. Rowing exercises are also good for Dysautonomia. Elevating the legs a little bit when you feel tired is good. You can even use a pillow to prop up your legs, when your blood pressure feels too low. Squiggling your toes from time to time will be of great help. Using compression stockings and leg weights will help with the condition.

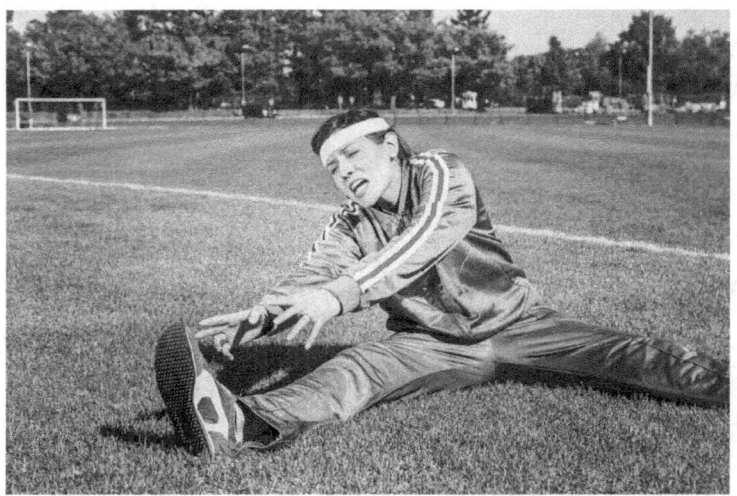

It is good to take short breaks in between work, instead of working long hours at a stretch. You should know your limits and pace yourself accordingly. It is better to take on one day at a time and not overdo things. It is important to rest and sleep well.

Be cautious while showering. It is better for you to take a bath sitting down in a chair, than standing up. You can probably use a showering chair for this.

This is a safe way of showering, especially on days when you feel beat up and exhausted.

You can adopt a regular routine of doing simple yoga exercises combined with meditation. This will help to relieve the stress and calm the mind. Guided visual imagery will help in getting a better result out of meditation.

You can take a massage therapy or acupuncture session to make the POTS Syndrome Dysautonomia better. This really depends on yourself and you have to be comfortable doing it. A massage with soothe and calm the nerves and reduce the stress.

You should eat 5 or 6 small meals in a day as opposed to 3 big meals. You should check for gluten allergy or lactose intolerance which usually affects people with Dysautonomia.

Keeping yourself cool is very important. It will be advisable to maintain an even temperature always. Heat is not helpful for POTS patients. So, try to keep cool and hydrated.

Do not isolate yourself. Try to be as socially active as your health allows. You might not be able to take part in late night parties; but you can surely enjoy a quiet evening with a few understanding friends. Seclusion will only lead to anxiety and depression and worsen the matters further. Get involved with friends, relatives and family as much as your heath permits, presently.

Take help. Do not hesitate to use the wheel chair when needed. When you go grocery shopping you could probably use the motorized shopping carts. Don't step back discerning about what others might think. Do not feel ashamed to make use of the help available at hand. Put your body and your well-being first.

Take up simple hobbies. No one can stop a person with POTS Syndrome Dysautonomia from reading books or watching movies! You can also play some board games and engage yourself as it does not involve much physical work. In fact, playing a game of chess can lift up your spirits and make you feel fresh and cool.

Prepare beforehand! It is always preferable to prepare yourself well before going out anywhere. Put all emergency requirements like a packet of chips, water and micro fan in a bag and keep it ready at all times.

Join a support group. It will be of great help to join a support group where you can meet other people who are similar to you and have identical symptoms. You can discuss with them and get new ideas about how to deal with the symptoms. It is also reassuring to see that there are others similar to us especially when we are in a shaky situation.

While the above tips and recommendations are generally useful, please select the ones which you feel most comfortable with. Further, remember that this book is only for general information and people should refer to doctor for medical advice.

Many people with the disease find it difficult to explain to others, what they are facing, because on the outside all looks pretty and well. Since this is a very rare condition, there is not much awareness about it. So, do not take the trouble of explaining too much to acquaintances. Instead you can just say that you have low blood pressure. That way, they will understand it better.

Even doctors may sometimes push you aside, because you do not present with a finite diagnosis. However, it is good to be assertive and frank with the doctors and be truthful with what you are experiencing. You can ask your doctor to prescribe some vitamins and supplements, which will help you.

Therefore, even if it is difficult to live with autonomia dysfunction, it is certainly not a deadly disease. It is a syndrome which can be managed well, by being smart. In the beginning, of course, the disease seems to be a little frightening with the sudden fainting spells and dizziness. However, when you get to know the specific ways in which it affects you, one will be able to successfully overcome the POTS Syndrome Dysautonomia. It is not a life threatening condition like heart attack, which might cause sudden death. You just have to take certain precautions in relation to diet and activities. If that is taken care of, you can enjoy a fulfilling life, despite the syndrome.

Wish you good luck!

One Last Thing...

If you enjoyed this book or found it useful, I'd be
very grateful if you'd post a short review on
Amazon.com
Your support really does make a difference and I
real all the reviews personally so, I can get your
feedback and make this book even better.
If you'd like to leave a review the all you need to do
is click the review link on this book's page on
Amazon.com

If you want to know the latest news and cures
about
Dysautonomia POTS Syndrome
Please LIKE my Facebook page at:

http://www.facebook.com/POTSSyndromeDisease